HOW WE
CONQUERED
KERATOCONUS

*First hand experiences from those who took back
their lives from their devastating eye disease*

Edited by
Brian S. Boxer Wachler, MD
World Leading Keratoconus Specialist
Foreword by Steven Holcomb, Olympic Gold Medalist

How We Conquered Keratoconus

For information about this title or to order other books and/or electronic
media, contact the publisher: .

Brian S. Boxer Wachler, MD, Inc., A Medical Corp
465 N. Roxbury Drive #902
Beverly Hills, CA 90210
310-860-1900
www.KeratoconusInserts.com
www.BoxerWachler.com
info@boxerwachler.com

ISBN: 978-0-615-63187-5

Printed in the United States of America

Please note individual results of any medical procedure will vary. To find out if you are a candidate or to have a complimentary record review, please contact:

Boxer Wachler Vision Institute
465 N. Roxbury Drive, Suite 902
Beverly Hills, CA 90210
phone: 310-860-1900
email: info@boxerwachler.com

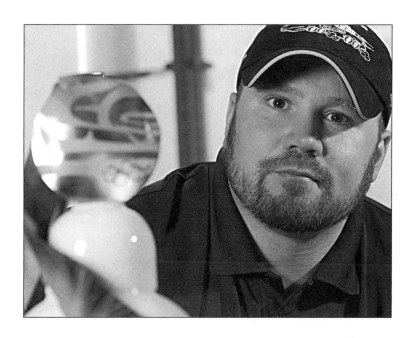

Foreword by Steven Holcomb,
Olympic Gold Medalist

I was diagnosed with Keratoconus sometime in the early 2000s. I can't pinpoint a date because, quite frankly, nobody could actually tell me if I had it or not. It's a disease that in its early stages can be difficult to diagnose. I was no different. I spent years bouncing around from one ophthalmologist to the next, changing my prescriptions and getting a second, a third, and fourth opinion. I ended up seeing twelve different doctors but still only had one prognosis: I would slowly go blind then have to have a cornea transplant. That was going to be my life and that is that, end of story.

Brian S. Boxer Wachler, MD

It was right after the 2006 Olympic Winter Games in Torino, Italy that I knew my life was over, at least as I saw it. Yes, cornea transplants are pretty standard these days and people manage to get by that way, but that wasn't what concerned me. My life was bobsledding. I had spent the better part of 8 years at that point working hard and climbing my way to the top of the sport in not only the United States but on the world class level. At 26 years old, I was the best bobsledder in the country, and on my way to being the best on the planet. All eyes were on me to win the next Olympic Medal for the United States. Everything I had worked so hard for, all the sacrifices I had made, the years of dedication and perseverance was about to be in vain, all because I couldn't read an eye chart.

It was late 2007 when I first heard about Dr. Brian and his C3-R procedure. A former bobsledder, now doctor, had mentioned to me that he had heard of a new procedure that may help my problem. He explained it a little and handed me a phone number. Now, at this point all I could think was, "I've seen 12 specialists, they all say there is no cure, and that a transplant is the only option. Yet, this guy, in Beverly Hills no less, is going to give me a few eye drops, I will stare at a light, and I'll be cured?" Now, obviously there is more to the science than just that. But on the surface that is exactly what it sounded like. Unfortunately, I was at a point in my life that it really didn't matter if it worked. I was either going to go stare at a light and be miraculously cured, or I wasn't. Either way, I had nothing to lose.

I finally met Dr. Brian on December 25, 2007. It was actually mid-season for me, and I was on my Christmas Break from bobsledding. I'm not sure if he knew who I was at the time, most people didn't, and since bobsledding is a pretty obscure sport compared to the professional leagues, I didn't really expect much. We talked quite a bit, and to be honest, it was a rather refreshing doctor visit. Again, I had been to 12 specialists before and heard nothing but bad news. This was different. There was a much different tone, a different feel about the conversation. When a doctor has a bad prognosis, no matter how mild, it was still bad news and there is just no way to hide it. There was always a tension in the air before. However it wasn't like that with Dr. Brian. He doesn't have bad news to give; he is there to finally give you good news and he knows it.

I went on to have the C3-R® procedure that very same day. It was completely painless other than the boredom of sitting there for 30 minutes. I didn't bring any music like I was told to, so I paid the consequences. Once it was over, Dr. Brian gave me some regular drops to keep my eyes moist and sent me on my way. I came in the following day for a post-procedure check-up, and everything was fine. I only say fine, because nothing was different. I was wearing the same contacts; I had no pain, no discomfort, no anything, as far as I could tell nothing happened. Either way, I made an appointment to come back in March after the bobsled season so we could work on correcting my vision. So I left and went back to what I do best, bobsledding.

My Keratoconus had progressed quite a bit over the last few years and I was getting a new prescription every 4 to 6 weeks. When I returned in March, I realized something that I was not expecting. It had been 13 weeks and I was still using the same lenses without an issue. In fact, I was actually seeing a tad bit better. I wouldn't have believed it myself if I didn't actually see it with my own eyes. It was amazing, maybe there *was* something to this C3-R®, and it actually worked. Could it really be that simple? It was.

I had the Visian ICL™ put in on March 6, 2008 and I went from 20/1000 to 20/20 in my right eye and 20/15 in my left. It was my first "Gold Medal", a second lease on life. One year later, almost to the day on March 1, 2009 I became the first American to win a Bobsled World Championship Title in 50 years. Nearly 2 years after my procedure on February 27, 2010 I was the first American to win an Olympic Gold Medal since 1948, that's a 62 year drought. Without my vision, none of that would have been possible.

I'm an Olympic Champion. I've been through the struggles, fought the fight on the playing field, and won. But before any of that, I struggled with, fought the fight and won against Keratoconus with the help of Dr. Brian. Before that my life was in a downward spiral. It didn't look good and I didn't have much time left. Definitely not enough to reach my full potential as an athlete and win more medals and world titles than any other American bobsledder. My meeting with Dr. Brian changed everything and I would not be here today without him.

I can sit here and tell you how great Dr. Brian is, how his C3-R® procedure changed my life, and how you should run out and get it done until I'm blue in the face. But all in all, one person doesn't matter. For all you know, maybe I just got lucky. Well, you're about to read story after story from individuals that have similar stories to mine, each one a success. The proof is in the pages.

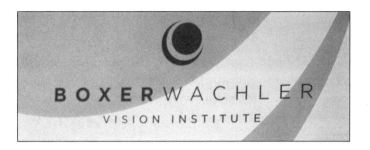

Introduction

Keratoconus is often a devastating and progressively worsening eye disease. There is a real, human side to every medical problem and it's no different with Keratoconus. Since the beginning of my career, I carefully listened to the countless stories of lives shattered by Keratoconus. Back then, the standard procedure was an invasive and painful cornea transplant.

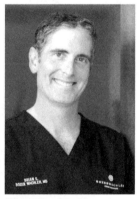

"Dr. Brian" S. Boxer Wachler

As a cornea surgeon I was routinely performing cornea transplants for Keratoconus early in my career, but I also was witnessing how difficult the recovery was for people, the complications, and how disruptive it was to their lives: 6 to 12 months to recover away from school, work, etc.

One night in 1999 I had a dream of developing something new for Keratoconus. People with Keratoconus needed a "physician advocate" as there really was not one. In 1999, I set out to be their advocate and invent new, less invasive treatments for Keratoconus. Many colleagues said to me, "Brian, corneal transplants work just fine. Don't waste your time."

Brian S. Boxer Wachler, MD

Not giving in to peer-pressure, I forged ahead and dedicated my career to inventing better procedures for people with Keratoconus. **In 1999, virtually no one had heard of Intacs® for Keratoconus when I started it.** I knew it was working. Physician colleagues said I should stop doing Intacs® and continue to do cornea transplants. But *I saw the happy patients with lives restored, the "fractures healed."* I continued to research and fine-tune Intacs® for Keratoconus so patients could avoid a corneal transplant. Perhaps that's the reason my work with Intacs® was not popular with my peers.

Now, all these years later, I am thrilled that Intacs® has become a main treatment for Keratoconus in our practice.

Even considering my success with Intacs® often dramatically improving vision, I recognized early on that Intacs® couldn't treat the underlying cause of Keratoconus, which is weakened collagen fibers in the cornea. **Thus, people with improved vision from Intacs® could still experience progression of their Keratoconus, therefore potentially worsening the improvements from Intacs®.** We needed a complementary procedure to stabilize the disease.

That's the reason in 2003 I began pioneering collagen crosslinking for Keratoconus and invented the *C3-R® Crosslinking System* which was designed to stabilize Keratoconus. I found that the process of using our proprietary Crosslinking Solution combined with a special ultraviolet light can NON-INVASIVELY stabilize Keratoconus. You'll read next how and why we changed the procedure name to Holcomb C3-R® after American bobsledder Steven Holcomb. **We also found the BEST results occur when Holcomb C3-R® is combined *with* Intacs® at the same time.**

Now all these years later **I am thrilled that my original dream has become reality for people with Keratoconus.** This book illustrates how lives can be restored and how many people conquered their own Keratoconus by refusing to accept their doctors' prison sentence of "you only have two options—hard contacts or cornea transplant." <u>It's finally a new era for Keratoconus treatments.</u>

Warmest regards,

Brian

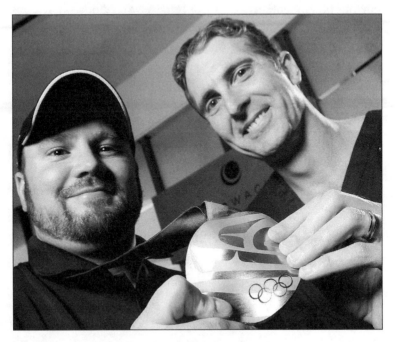

The Historic Steven Holcomb Story . . . From Blindness to Olympic Gold

Since he was a kid growing up in Park City, Utah, *Steven Holcomb dreamed of Olympic gold* and it wasn't long before he learned to tame the power and speed of one of the world's most dangerous sports: bobsledding. Steven climbed up the ranks of bobsled drivers and led the United States to solid finishes in the 2006 Olympic Games. The future was bright. *But in 2007 a potentially blinding eye disease changed everything.*

Steven explained, "I was diagnosed with Keratoconus. My eyes started to degenerate over time. In 2007 I was at the point where either I was going to lose my vision or have a cornea transplant. And either way it was going to put me out

of the sport." Dreams of Olympic gold could be gone forever. Steven was devastated, but took one last chance when his team doctor sent him to Dr. Brian for C3-R®. After C3-R® treated his Keratoconus, insertable lenses were placed behind Steven's iris, restoring Steven's vision to 20/20 and giving him a chance to make an amazing comeback.

After the procedure Steven said, "Once you're able to see, things open up again—you're a lot more confident. I can go out there and drive and use my skills the way that they're meant to be used." <u>In Steven's case, his skills were used to earn the United States its first Olympic gold medal in bobsledding in 62 years</u>. Steven explained, "I've focused on winning a gold medal since I was a kid and to actually be sitting here with a gold medal is kind of unreal."

Dr. Brian explained, "As soon as Steven and his team were announced as the winners of the gold, my emotions just overtook me. I was sobbing, tears streaming down my face. I was hugging everybody." But even more powerful was the response from the American public and from people all over the world who wrote thousands of emails and letters to share how Steven's story inspired them to reach new heights of their own.

Steven says, "I was given a 'second chance' and now SO MANY other people can have a 'second chance' with these procedures that Dr. Brian has performed almost daily since 2003 for patients coming from around the world."

Due to the worldwide recognition Steven brought to the C3-R® procedure, it was renamed "Holcomb C3-R®" on *The Doctors* TV show on April 9, 2010. *This marked the first time a procedure was named in honor of an Olympic athlete.* Steven and Holcomb C3-R® are now world famous.

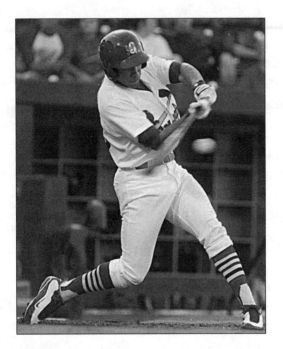

Tommy Pham

As a baseball player for the Cardinals, I noticed my vision quickly got bad a couple of years ago. My manager suggested that I should get my eyes checked. I went to the mall, a little local eye doctor, and got some glasses prescribed to me. Throughout the season I wore those glasses. I didn't feel that they were really helping. I was still striking out a lot, so I ditched them. After the season in 2009 my director suggested that I go to St. Louis and see our team eye doctor. That's when I was diagnosed with early Keratoconus.

Since 2009 I've been wearing gas permeable contacts, which helped me see better and helped my hitting and my reaction time to the ball from the outfield. Then I realized how important vision is to what I do as a baseball player.

Unfortunately my vision started to get worse even with the gas permeable contact lenses. Things started appearing blurry all over again. It was getting harder for me to read things and visually process things. The nightmare was returning. I was told a BIG MYTH that gas permeable contact lenses hold back the Keratoconus. They don't—the Keratoconus just gets worse and worse and you have to keep getting new contacts to keep pace with the deterioration.

Thankfully I was told that the Holcomb C3-R® from Dr. Brian was very beneficial and could stop the Keratoconus. *From my research, Dr. Brian is not only the best Keratoconus doctor in the world, but he also cares about his patients.* You can't put a price on that "world champion" combination.

After the Holcomb C3-R® procedure I was surprised that it really was a **pain-free experience** and I was back to 100% of my normal activities the next day and even put my contacts back in. I've been through "real deal" surgery twice before and I've come out crying from the pain. Here, with the Holcomb C3-R® you are in the super cushy chair, relaxed, feet kicked up for 30 minutes. And you're done. It's a pretty relaxing experience. They treat you very good here. That is always a plus too. **Thank you Dr. Brian for saving my baseball career!**

—Tommy Pham, baseball player
Intacs® and Holcomb C3-R® in 2011

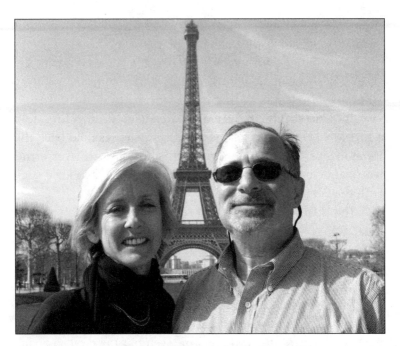

Physician-Patient Enjoys Many Years of Continued Stability after Holcomb C3-R®!

As a doctor, when I first noticed something out of kilter with my sight I went to the optometrist and got glasses. I never got used to my glasses and stopped wearing them. About 2 years later, *I began to get progressively more annoyed with the distortion in my left eye.* I was again told I had astigmatism, got glasses, grew tired of them, stopped wearing them, and stopped thinking about it.

Another 4 years passed and one evening, as <u>I was driving home from work, I noticed that I could barely read the street signs due to incredible distortion and fuzziness.</u> I WAS FREAKED OUT TO SAY THE LEAST. I went to my ophthalmologist who looked at me, ran some tests and told me I had Keratoconus. I did some research and learned that I had <u>an essentially incurable and progressive condition that would result in legal blindness and corneal transplants</u>.

I went to the local optometrist and got fitted with special Keratoconus tailored contact lenses. But I COULD NEVER TOLERATE HARD LENSES and so they went the way of my glasses—into the drawer, remaining unused. I tried soft lenses, same thing.

During this ordeal, I learned about Dr. Brian and Intacs® with Holcomb C3-R®. At the time it seemed very experimental, yet encouraging. Dr. Brian advised me to receive both Holcomb C3-R® and Intacs®. I had the operation about seven years ago.

<u>I have essentially a normal life and have experienced, rather than progression, a significant improvement.</u> I would like to thank Dr. Brian for the priceless gift he has given me, my sight!

—Howard D. Epstein, MD in Southern California
Intacs® and Holcomb C3-R® in 2005

**Know Your Treatment Options—Have a
COMPLIMENTARY Record Review by Dr. Brian**

1. Request a copy of your most recent eye exam
with color cornea maps from your doctor

2. Describe your situation on a cover sheet with the
best phone number and email to contact you

3. Scan and email to: info@boxerwachler.com, or mail to:

Boxer Wachler Vision Institute—KC Records Review
465 N. Roxbury Drive, Suite 902
Beverly Hills, CA 90210

**If you have questions, please call us at 310-860-1900.
After Dr. Brian's review, we will contact to discuss.**

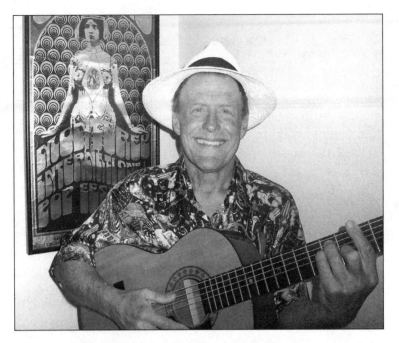

Conquering the Keratoconus Blues

The Keratoconus Blues by Don Basseri

V1

G   C G
Dr. Boxer Wachler, it's an odd name to say,

     A7 D
yet he was the one who rose up, to save the day.

G   C G
He gave me hope when my future wasn't clear,

      D   G

that innovative Dr. B is always welcome around here.

V2

G   C   G

A7   D

Going blind is a scary thing, it can make a grown man cry,
when the signs on the road disappear before your very eyes.

G   C

G   D

He's got a simple procedure, and it worked like a magic trick,

    G

If I had to come up with a man of the year, Dr. B would be my pick.

V3

G   C   G

A7   D

All the other doctors said there was nothing they could do,
the sad compassion in their eyes just added to my Blues.

G   C   G

The gift of sight means more than anything I can say,

           D   G

with Dr. B's creative touch I'm thankful every day.

—Don Basseri, Northern California
Holcomb C3-R® in 2008

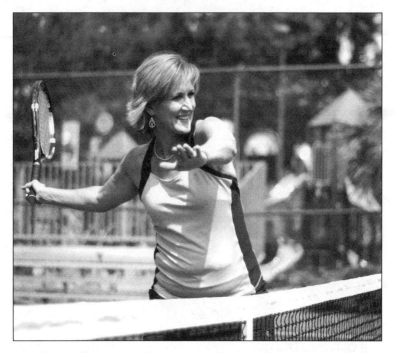

Cornea Transplant? Not for Me!!

If you feel there is no hope, be encouraged because <u>there is HOPE!</u> Keratoconus is a disease that a lot of people do not know even exists. I was one of those people. In my 20s I was diagnosed with Keratoconus, which started a long and frustrating journey of trial and error—trying to find something that would work. *I can remember how hopeless I felt.*

After trying many contacts, the doctor basically told me that the best option I had was a cornea transplant. I didn't know what to do and was not informed of any other options. **I finally decided to find the best doctor to perform the surgery by searching "Keratoconus" and I discovered Dr. Brian.**

I began to read his website and found that there was another option. I sent my eye records in for him to review and he found that I was a candidate for Intacs® and Holcomb C3-R®.

I flew out to California and Dr. Brian performed Intacs® and Holcomb C3-R® to reverse and stabilize the Keratoconus and improve my eyesight. <u>I was so excited and relieved that I didn't have to have the cornea transplant</u>!

I continued to keep up with Dr. Brian and all of the amazing procedures available for Keratoconus patients and four years later I had Visian ICL™ done. *Now I do not have to wear contacts at all!* I can truly say that <u>Dr.Brian helped me to begin life again.</u>

We cannot put a price on our sight; it affects everything we do! Thank you Dr. Brian for your diligent study in inventing techniques and procedures to help Keratoconus patients like myself find HOPE again! I am forever grateful!

—Kay Kisser, Florida
Intacs® and Holcomb C3-R® in 2005
Visian ICL in 2009

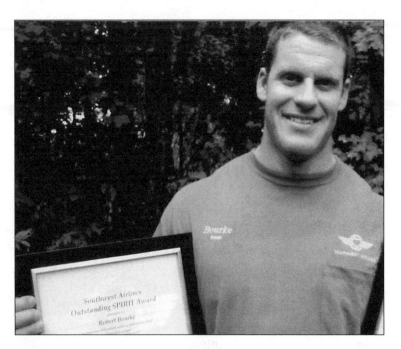

Bobby Bourke

Bobby was living life in a blur. He had to hold his cell phone within two inches of his nose to make a call or text a message. He would have to sit two feet away from the TV in the living room. He couldn't recognize people, even friends, who were just 10 feet away.

Then Bobby and his wife Cassi watched Steven Holcomb at the 2010 Winter Olympics in Vancouver win Gold. Cassi did her research which led her and Bobby to Dr. Brian. He performed Holcomb C3-R®, Intacs®, and CK. To say Bobby got a new lease on life would be an understatement. The following letter from his parents says what routinely occurs after Dr. Brian helps people with Keratoconus.

DR. BRIAN:
Hello! Enclosed is a photo of Bobby Bourke, our son, and one of your successful keratoconus patients. He's holding a "certificate of completion" and an "outstanding spirit award" for his new job at Southwest Airlines. He is a "ramp agent", one of those guys you see moving luggage, guiding in the planes with those lights they hold and pushing the plane out with those little, but very powerful little cars. He loves his new job. And we don't think it would be possible if we hadn't heard about you & gotten the treatment he needed. He can be a productive asset to society ~~entirely~~ instead of ending up on disability, which he would have HATED. We can not thank you enough! You are truly our hero!

                    Bob + Rhonda Bourke

                    Industry PA 15052

Thank you a million times!

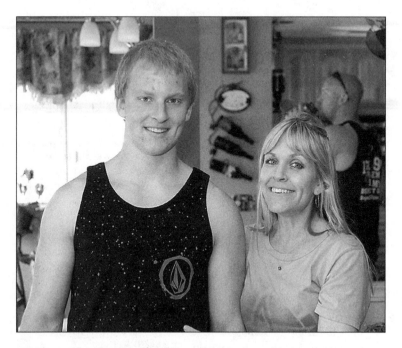

Holcomb C3-R® Rescues Teenager!

My son Connor was fifteen years old when he first started struggling to see. It didn't really sink in until we took him to get his driving permit. He failed the eye exam and was told that he probably needed glasses. <u>A week later Connor was diagnosed with Keratoconus, and informed that a cornea transplant might be in his future.</u>

For some, prescription glasses can help, but Connor needed to wear rigid hard glass lenses. We started going to appointments almost weekly because it was so difficult to fit Connor with lenses. His vision was soon 20/70 and worsening. Connor was referred to a specialist in Keratoconus fittings and she was able to get a prescription that fit well.

Then we came across Steven Holcomb's story. We were inspired and excited. I decided to do some research and learned that Holcomb C3-R® could keep him from deteriorating further. I talked with all of his eye care professionals about the procedure, and they encouraged us to pursue it. I sent Connor's records in for Dr. Brian to review and he determined he was a candidate for Holcomb C3-R®.

I scheduled the appointment for the Holcomb C3-R® about eight months after Connor's initial diagnosis. It has now been several months since his C3-R®, and he is doing excellent! HIS EYES HAVE STOPPED IN THEIR TRACKS.

We were at the eye doctor almost every week when we found out he had Keratoconus, and we felt hopeless doing nothing to keep his eyes from rapidly worsening. **The Holcomb C3-R® gave us the option to arrest this disease** and we are very thankful to Dr. Brian for making this possible.

—Becky, Connor's Mother, Northern California
Holcomb C3-R® in 2010

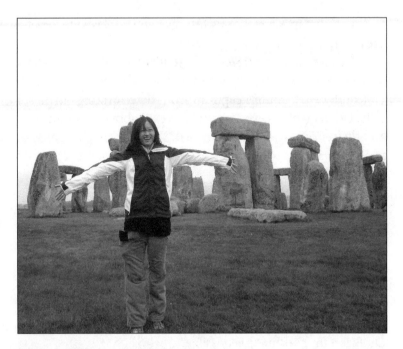

Local Doctor Told Her "Keratoconus Not Curable"

I always knew there was something wrong with my eyes. When I was four years old, I was already in glasses. I felt my vision varied day-by-day, hour by hour. I started to wear RGP (Rigid Gas Permeable) lenses when I was 22, but I wanted to correct my vision.

I knew I wasn't a candidate for laser surgery because of my unstable eyes but I couldn't resist getting a consultation. It was at that appointment that <u>I found out what was wrong with my eyes—Keratoconus. It was liberating and depressing at the same time.</u> Liberating because I finally knew what was wrong, but depressing because the doctor made it clear that this was progressive and said, **"Keratoconus is not curable,"** and "there are limited treatments that would only delay the inevitable." I felt desperate for an alternative of any kind.

Then I met a woman named Dolores who had Keratoconus and had it treated successfully! She recommended me to Dr. Brian who performed her surgery. Feeling a little desperate, I decided to go to Beverly Hills for the Holcomb C3-R® procedure.

When I went in for the initial exam and consultation, Dr. Brian asked me about my hopes and I replied: "I would really like to see without glasses or contacts but if that can't be helped, at least stop my eyes from getting worse!" He acknowledged my hopes and told me there was a procedure that would give me a 50% chance of seeing 20/20. On my 27th birthday I was seeing 20/20 without glasses or contacts. It was a dream come true! I couldn't be happier!

—Alice Tsai, Southern California
Holcomb C3-R® and Visian ICL in 2009

Know Your Treatment Options—Have a COMPLIMENTARY Record Review by Dr. Brian

1. Request a copy of your most recent eye exam with color cornea maps from your doctor

2. Describe your situation on a cover sheet with the best phone number and email to contact you

3. Scan and email to: info@boxerwachler.com, or mail to:

Boxer Wachler Vision Institute—KC Records Review
465 N. Roxbury Drive, Suite 902
Beverly Hills, CA 90210

If you have questions, please call us at 310-860-1900. After Dr. Brian's review, we will contact to discuss.

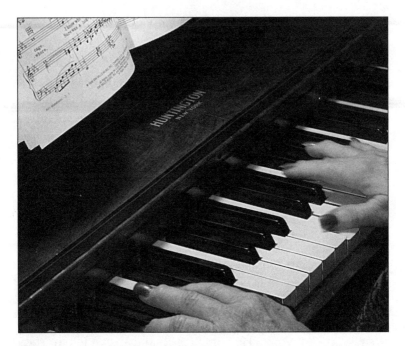

Fifteen Years of Struggle Come to an End!

At the age of 40 I was diagnosed with bilateral Keratoconus by my ophthalmologist, who referred me for evaluation to a Corneal Transplant Specialist as my only hope for treatment. I was devastated. **For 5 years the cone on my corneas deteriorated rapidly.**

After using gas permeable hard lenses for some time, the Keratoconus stopped and transplants were not needed for the time being. Then I was prescribed Saturn soft contact lenses with a hard center. I soon began rejecting them and experiencing frequent corneal lesions. After more than 15 years of this

PAINFUL experience with my corneas, <u>I learned about a new surgical procedure being done to correct Keratoconus.</u>

After some inquiries, I got in contact with Dr. Brian who thought I was a good candidate for Intacs®. I came into his office for corneal tests, and the next day had the surgery. Following a very short recovery, I went to have breakfast and I COULD READ THE SMALL LETTERS on a marmalade jar without any lenses at all!

I was fitted with soft contact lenses and prescription eye glasses, but even without them I can get around the house without any problem. Before, I could only see the silhouettes and shadows of nearby objects without wearing glasses. <u>I had the surgery five and a half years ago, and my life has changed and improved greatly</u> since that day! I want to take this opportunity to express again my deep gratitude to Dr. Brian.

—Clara G. Navarro, Mexico
Intacs® and Holcomb C3-R® in 2005

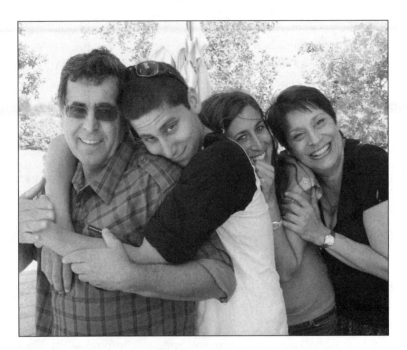

My Son was Diagnosed with Keratoconus

When my son was 14 years old we received notification from his school that his routine eye exam showed a problem and that we needed to consult with an ophthalmologist. We went to see one and were told that he had Keratoconus. I took my son to our optometrist, thinking he just needed glasses. Our optometrist immediately realized the problem and sat us down to explain what Keratoconus was, what could happen, and what options we had.

He handed me a list of experts in the field and told us the "good news" was that if it worsened, he could always get a corneal transplant. <u>I went on the computer and began to research</u>

Keratoconus. I came across a site that described a new technique called Holcomb C3-R®. *Within a week we made an appointment with Dr. Brian.*

My son was not the calmest or quietest of boys, yet when they painted the Crosslinking Solution on his corneas and shone the light onto them, he was still and cooperative. **He felt no pain or any discomfort afterward.** We were told that he was their youngest patient so they didn't know how effective the treatment would be on him but, if needed, he could have the treatment again in the future.

It's been seven years and every single appointment he has had has been the same—absolutely stable! As a mother, being able to find the solution and help my son keep his vision was the best reward. His life is as normal as everyone else around him. I couldn't wish for anything more than that!

—Dina Golan, Tal's Mother, Israel
Holcomb C3-R® in 2005

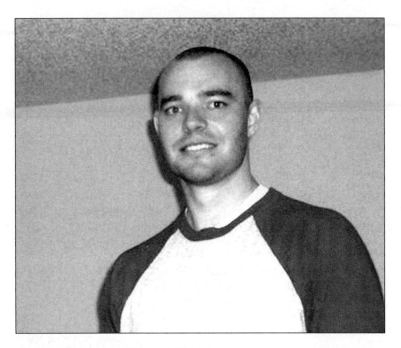

Keratoconus after LASIK

In 2001 I had laser surgery, and then about seven years later I found that I had something wrong in my right eye. Doctors told me that I had an eye disease called Keratoconus in my right eye. I am still not sure if my eye problem was a result of the laser surgery or from Keratoconus.

I was a little worried because I didn't know anything about Keratoconus or how it would affect my vision, so I decided to do some research. **I found Dr. Brian's website, and read up on his procedures and surgeries.** <u>I was definitely glad to know that there were some options out there and that I was not alone.</u>

I requested that Dr. Brian review my eye records to see what I would be a candidate for.

In March 2010, I was able to get the Holcomb C3-R®, Intacs®, and CK procedures from Dr. Brian. I was a little nervous at first, but all of the procedures went well. I felt very relaxed and comfortable throughout each procedure and when I was done I was very glad that I went ahead with all three of the treatments.

About a month later I was able to try out contacts in my right eye. <u>I can definitely tell a big difference in my vision</u> with the contacts. I feel pretty lucky to have improved my vision as much as I did with the help of Dr. Brian. IT'S HELPED IMPROVE MY EVERYDAY LIFE FROM WORK TO PLAYING BASKETBALL WITH FRIENDS.

I feel very lucky that I went through with the procedures.

—Bryon Lukso, Arizona
Intacs®, CK and Holcomb C3-R® in 2010

Brian S. Boxer Wachler, MD

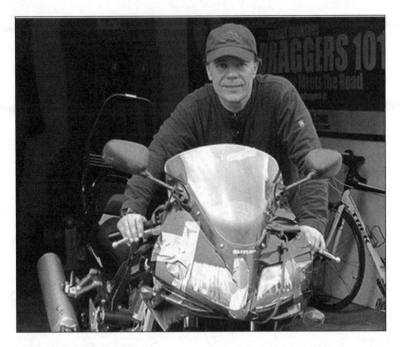

Gave Me Freedom!

I've had Keratoconus for about 10 years. For years my Keratoconus condition denied me the ability to wear contact lenses. Sports, motorcycling, biking, martial arts and even my work activities required numerous pairs of glasses. **I longed for freedom from my glasses.**

Recently, I was informed that a crosslinking study was being started in the Washington D.C. area, where I live. I considered applying, but after research and careful consideration I realized that I would be better served by going to the renowned surgeon who had pioneered the technique and Dr. Brian performed a record review from my eye doctor here in Virginia.

The experience and results were well worth the 2,700 mile flight!

<u>The results were better than I expected, and the staff is the best I've ever experienced</u>. I felt confident in the professional abilities of each office member I came in contact with. The best part was the warm personable aspects and kindness of the staff that treated you like family. **The results of the Holcomb C3-R®, Intacs® and CK are that I can comfortably wear a contact lens in my treated right eye, when before I could not.**

My near vision has also improved and I'm 40+ years old. <u>I now am experiencing the freedom I waited for</u> *and am able to better participate in the activities I enjoy so much.* **Even if you live a great distance away, Dr. Brian and his staff keep in touch with you,** are responsive to your concerns or questions, and make you feel like a member of their family, this has been my experience.

—Chris Medvigy, Virginia
Intacs®, CK, and Holcomb C3-R® in 2010

Know Your Treatment Options—Have a COMPLIMENTARY Record Review by Dr. Brian

1. Request a copy of your most recent eye exam with color cornea maps from your doctor

2. Describe your situation on a cover sheet with the best phone number and email to contact you

3. Scan and email to: info@boxerwachler.com, or mail to:
Boxer Wachler Vision Institute—KC Records Review
465 N. Roxbury Drive, Suite 902
Beverly Hills, CA 90210

If you have questions, please call us at 310-860-1900. After Dr. Brian's review, we will contact to discuss.

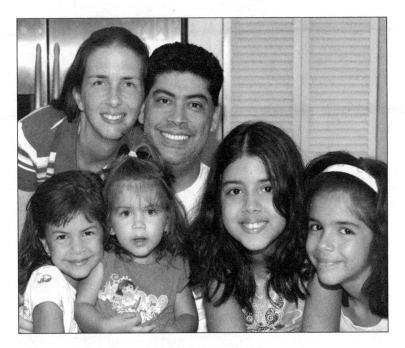

Changing Prescriptions Stopped!

A t age 5, I got my first pair of glasses. As I got older they became a nuisance and I began looking for an alternative. Contacts seemed to be the answer. After a while I was trying to find yet another solution. Then I heard about LASIK. I was quick to sign up for the procedure. I received the results I had been longing for.

Unfortunately, I only enjoyed perfect vision for about three months then needed glasses again. THE ASTIGMATISM GOT WORSE versus my original myopia. <u>My prescription was constantly changing. Then, I was diagnosed with Keratoconus.</u> *The countdown to a cornea transplant had begun.*

Out of desperation, I turned to the Internet for a Keratoconus solution and this lead me to Dr. Brian. Before booking my flight I was interested to see what he thought, so I sent in my eye exam records. <u>To my relief, he told me he was indeed able to help and within weeks I boarded a plane to Beverly Hills.</u> I clearly remember when Dr. Brian asked me what my goals were in regard to my vision. Without hesitation, I answered to save my corneas.

After the Holcomb C3-R® procedure, meeting Dr. Brian and realizing what a competent physician he is, I immediately felt comfortable and trusted my eyes to him. Dr. Brian recommended that I could enhance my vision by having Intacs®.

Thanks to Dr. Brian I no longer have to worry about a cornea transplant and enjoy much improved vision—Dr. Brian is the only person I trust to help me obtain 20/20 vision.

—Ernesto Perez, Florida
Intacs®, Holcomb C3-R® & PRK in 2008

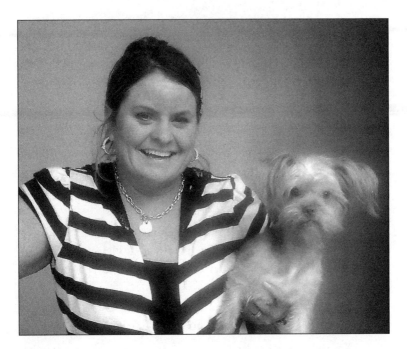

I Escaped the Curse of Painful Contact Lenses

I was diagnosed with Keratoconus in 1999. <u>As a patient you don't know to ask about things you have no idea exist</u>. NO ONE mentioned any options for me except eventual cornea transplant. <u>I was terrified of rejecting transplants.</u>

After 4 years of glasses, I was told my vision could no longer be corrected. Then I met a Keratoconus specialist who fitted me for KC contact lenses. I proceeded to go through several types until one day the lenses were causing excruciating pain. My worst nightmare was realized. My right eye needed a transplant. I frantically started searching for an alternative and came across Dr. Brian's website.

On my next visit to the corneal specialist my hopes were crushed as I was told to dismiss the idea of Holcomb C3-R®. **A while later, a friend called me raving about Steven Holcomb and how he had gotten his Keratoconus treated by a doctor in Beverly Hills.** After realizing it was Dr. Brian, I knew I had found a way out.

My right eye was beyond repair and I had my transplant. Then I saw Dr. Brian to have my left eye evaluated. <u>After receiving Holcomb C3-R® I no longer live in fear of the progression of Keratoconus in my left eye</u>! THAT ALONE HAS NO PRICE TAG.

I am able to wear a lens and have had no problems whatsoever. I finally feel free! I am so grateful for the knowledge that Dr. Brian has. Without him I would have had not one transplant but two.

Thank you Dr. Brian and staff, you do make a difference.

—Amy Beth Bryan, Southern California
Holcomb C3-R® in 2010

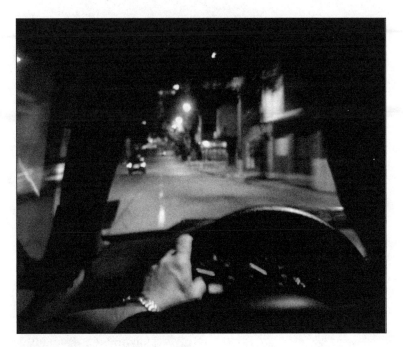

Now I Can Drive at Night

Que tal yo tenia un problema de queratocono mas pronunciado en el ojo izquierdo, se me practico la operación poniéndome Intacs®, dicha operación a mi me ayudo a mejorar mi vista ya que antes de esta yo no distinguía letras chicas a distancia y después si las puedo ver con facilidad esto es lo que se refiere el ojo Izquierdo, <u>yo tenia un problema cuando conducía de noche siempre terminaba mareado,</u> y con esta operación lo supere por completo ahora puedo manejar las horas que sean y no me mareo. <u>Por esto le doy las gracias al doctor bóxer por haberme ayuda a corregir mi vista y a superar del mareo cuando conduzco de noche.</u>

English Translation:

My Keratoconus was more pronounced in my left eye. I underwent Intacs® which helped my vision. Before I wasn't able to distinguish small print at a distance, but now I am able to. I used to have trouble driving at night because I always ended up dizzy and with this surgery I was able to overcome that completely. I'm able to drive many hours without feeling dizzy. This is why **I give many thanks to Dr. Brian for being able to help correct my vision and help me overcome my dizziness from driving at night.**

—Ignacio de la Rocha Cruz, Southern California
Intacs® and Holcomb C3-R® in 2009

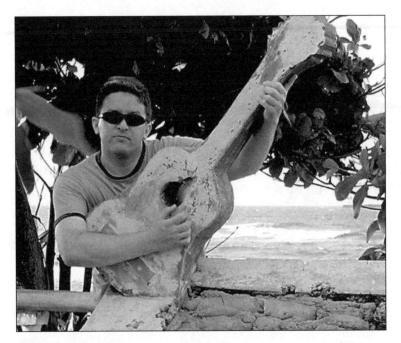

Worth Every Dollar that I Spent Because I No Longer Live in Fear of Needing a Transplant!

A t age of 26 I was diagnosed with Keratoconus. As my eyes worsened I tried several different lenses to the point where there was nothing else I could do but get a cornea transplant.

Then I decided to get further educated about Keratoconus through the Internet. I realized that I was not alone, but there were a lot of people much worse off than I was. I felt grateful for where I was and that it wasn't worse. At the same time it seemed like I had done everything that I could and that the next item was a cornea transplant, yet that seemed like too big of a leap. There HAD to be something in between what I had and a transplant.

Then I found it. I discovered Dr. Brian. This was what I was looking for. I read over everything, watched the videos, and contacted his office. I had to budget to pay for the procedure, but <u>if it halted the progression of my Keratoconus, wouldn't that be worth it</u>? Taking a corneal transplant out of the equation forever would be worth the budgeting.

I was nervous. With any medical procedure there are always risks, but *THIS ONE seemed like a no-brainer.* I scheduled an appointment and booked a flight to Los Angeles. The first thing I noticed about Dr. Brian and his staff was how *un*-Beverly Hills they were. They were very friendly, down-to-earth, and patient in answering every question; TOP NOTCH in all aspects.

The procedure was easier than I expected. After the procedure I went to the hotel and slept. The next day was a follow-up and then I was on my way back home. The procedures were <u>absolutely worth every dollar I spent, I no longer live in fear.</u>

When I go to the eye doctor, I no longer get those pangs of fear wondering "how much has it changed now" or "how much closer is the transplant". **My left eye hasn't had any vision changes since I had Holcomb C3-R® in 2007.** That's five years of the same prescription! I'm still at 20/20. <u>It truly is a gift, and the main reason for that gift is Dr. Brian.</u> <u>Not only is he a great doctor, but he really cares about his patients and his staff.</u>

<u>If there's anything I regret at this point, I wish I would have heard about Dr. Brian much earlier.</u> But since I didn't maybe you can. <u>You don't have to live in fear.</u> <u>There is hope!</u> The technology exists!

—Collin Johnson, Texas
Holcomb C3-R® in 2007

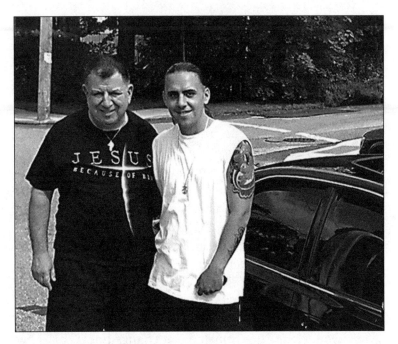

Botched Intacs® Surgery Elsewhere Fixed by Dr. Brian

I had been having blurry, distorted vision for about one year when I was diagnosed with Keratoconus at age 15. *I worried that I would NEVER have a normal life and eventually go blind.*

After a lot of research I found Dr. Brian's great website, but decided to first go to a highly regarded doctor near my home for Intacs® surgery. Unfortunately, the operation didn't go as planned. After making the incision something went wrong with the equipment and he was unable to put the Intacs® in. Months later when my eye had healed from the failed surgery, the doctor wanted to operate again. But I felt uncomfortable after what happened the first time. In my heart I knew I wanted Dr. Brian to do it, but the cost was too much for my family.

Dr. Brian provided me with a complimentary review of my records and determined that he could fix the problems. <u>With the help of my church I was able to have Dr. Brian do it</u>. His staff was so nice and made me feel at ease. Dr. Brian explained my options and I went ahead with Intacs®, CK, and Holcomb C3-R®.

Last year I PASSED MY DRIVER'S LICENSE TEST! I see pretty well now without glasses and can wear soft contacts. I would like to thank Dr. Brian and his staff for their excellent care, truly a great doctor and staff. I thank my family who were instrumental in my healing, my church, and most of all God. Like the song, <u>"I once was blind but now I see."</u>

—Giancarlo Murillo, New York
Intacs®, CK and Holcomb C3-R® in 2008

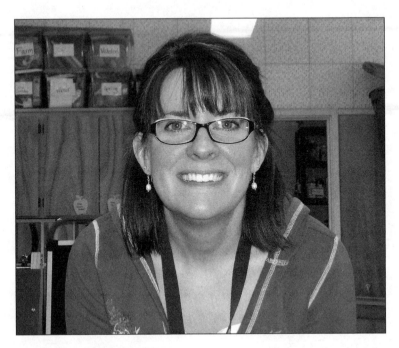

It Was a Miracle!

In 2006 I noticed that my distance vision was not as clear as it had been. In fact, it was now at the point that I had to squint to see clearly. I went to a local eye doctor who referred me to a corneal specialist and was diagnosed with Keratoconus. I had several follow-up appointments with the specialists and was informed that I would eventually need a corneal transplant.

There was, however, a doctor in Beverly Hills who had invented a procedure that I might be a candidate for. **The decision was not "if" I would have surgery—rather what type of surgery I would have.**

In 2008, after doing exhaustive research on my own, I decided to contact Dr. Brian. I made an appointment and went to see him. He and his staff were genuinely caring and kind. Dr. Brian determined that I was a good candidate for Intacs®, Holcomb C3-R®, and CK. Dr. Brian stated that due to my intolerance of a contact lens to correct my vision, this surgery, aside from a corneal transplant, was my only option.

I had the surgery and the next morning I was amazed to find that only one day after surgery I could already see functionally in both eyes. *It was a miracle!* It has been just over four years since my successful surgery with Dr. Brian. MY VISION IS STABLE and I AM HAPPILY ABLE TO WEAR GLASSES for minimal vision correction.

I am forever thankful to Dr. Brian!

—Gretchen Gooby, Arizona
Intacs®, CK and Holcomb C3-R® in 2008

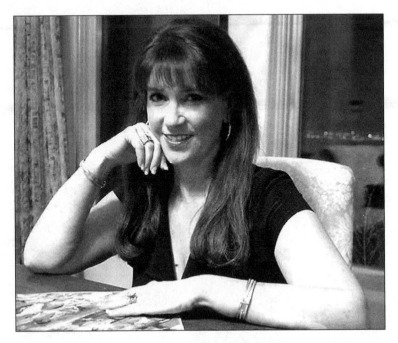

Yeah! Now I Can Wear Soft Contact Lenses!

Fifteen years ago I was diagnosed with Keratoconus. The only treatments available were hard contact lenses and corneal transplants. My ophthalmologist told me to hang in there because in the future there would probably be some kind of procedure for Keratoconus, but he did not know what or when.

I was fit with hard contact lenses and I would see well with them, but IT WAS DIFFICULT WEARING HARD LENSES. I was later fitted with Synergeyes lenses. They were comfortable and I had 20/20 vision with them until they would fog up.

Feeling desperate, I began researching for any possible therapy for Keratoconus and found Dr. Brian. I went back to my ophthalmologist and he told me that <u>I had reached the point where I would need a corneal transplant</u>. However, **my eye doctor in New Mexico mentioned Holcomb C3-R® as my best option and recommended Dr. Brian.** Dr. Brian agreed after reviewing my records and advised about the possibility of Intacs® and CK to provide additional improvement in my vision.

I traveled to Beverly Hills and met Dr. Brian and his staff. It was an incredibly wonderful and comfortable experience. They were all very knowledgeable and caring. I had the Intacs®, Holcomb C3-R®, and the CK procedures done. The procedures were certainly not difficult and for the first time ever, I truly had hope.

I AM NOW ABLE TO WEAR SOFT CONTACT LENSES AND ACTUALLY SEE OUT OF THEM! I cannot begin to tell you how grateful I am for this opportunity and to Dr. Brian and his staff for making the experience pleasant and possible.

—Esther Davis, Ph.D., New Mexico
Intacs®, CK and Holcomb C3-R® in 2010

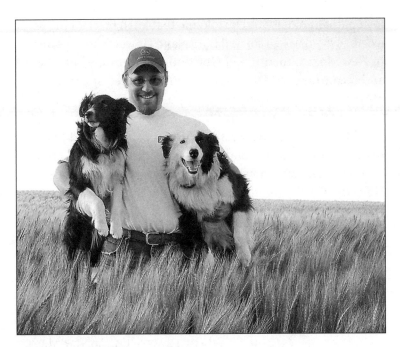

I Got My Life Back From Keratoconus!

When I was 14 years old I was diagnosed with Keratoconus. <u>I was told my only option to treat it was hard contact lenses.</u> My eyes were always irritated and I rubbed my eyes a lot, which only made my condition worse.

Eventually I stopped wearing the contacts and just lived with the poor vision. Fast forward 10 years and I needed a commercial driver's license. *The only way I could get one was to have 20/40 vision in each eye, so back to the contacts I went.*

I soon remembered why I quit wearing them the first time and decided it was time to find an alternative. I was looking on the Internet when I stumbled across the Boxer Wachler Vision

Institute and Holcomb C3-R® procedure, which intrigued me. I sent Dr. Brian my eye exam records to review. **Several months later I found myself in California visiting Dr. Brian and his staff.** I had Intacs®, CK, and the Holcomb C3-R® procedures done.

It has now been three years since the surgery and my eyes have completely stabilized and my corrected vision with glasses is 20/20 and 20/25. <u>I can now hold my commercial driver's license and day-to-day operations are so much more enjoyable</u>. I can see what I am doing and I can also do it in comfort. I no longer worry that simply mowing the lawn could cause me severe irritation and pain.

<u>This surgery Dr. Brian performed gave me my life back</u> and I am very grateful to him and his staff for providing an alternative to the traditional treatments for this disease.

—Mike Ladenburg, Montana
Intacs®, CK and Holcomb C3-R® in 2009

Know Your Treatment Options—Have a COMPLIMENTARY Record Review by Dr. Brian

1. Request a copy of your most recent eye exam with color cornea maps from your doctor

2. Describe your situation on a cover sheet with the best phone number and email to contact you

3. Scan and email to: info@boxerwachler.com, or mail to:

Boxer Wachler Vision Institute—KC Records Review
465 N. Roxbury Drive, Suite 902
Beverly Hills, CA 90210

If you have questions, please call us at 310-860-1900.
After Dr. Brian's review, we will contact to discuss.

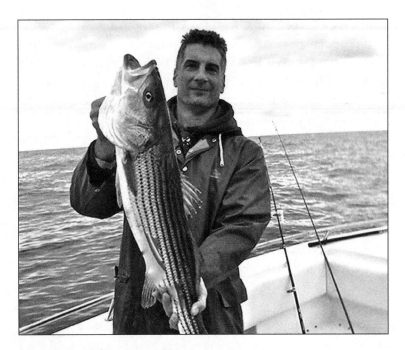

Past Day-to-Day Challenges Now Completely Erased!

When I was diagnosed with Keratoconus <u>I was told that there was no cure</u> and the disease usually levels off with age.

I lived the next 10 years with inconsistent, blurred vision. <u>Upon turning 40 with no signs of the disease slowing down I began to have major concerns.</u> On my own I started to research and came across Dr. Brian's website. This was <u>the first time in 12 years that I felt a glimmer of hope</u>.

I booked an appointment and had my eye doctor chart sent in for Dr. Brian to review. He determined I would likely benefit from Intacs®, CK and Holcomb C3-R®. Upon my visit, the first thing that struck me was the positive and knowledgeable atmosphere. The attention the staff gave me made me feel at ease. I was a candidate for both Holcomb C3-R® and Intacs®. **Dr. Brian explained in great detail the exact steps and expectations of the procedures.**

I returned the following day and after a few hours all was complete. There was <u>no</u> pain and the recovery went exactly as Dr. Brian explained it would. IT'S BEEN ALMOST TWO YEARS AND MY VISION IS MORE STABLE AND CLEARER THAN IN THE PAST 20 YEARS. All of the day-to-day challenges I lived with have been completely erased. <u>My quality of living has been raised to a level I thought I would never experience again</u>.

A day hasn't gone by that I have not counted my blessings for finding Dr. Brian and his amazing treatments to help me fight Keratoconus. <u>He believed there was hope when all others didn't.</u>

—Jeff Gagliotti, New York
Intacs®, CK and Holcomb C3-R® in 2010

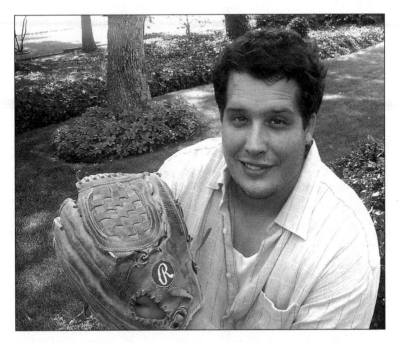

Shocked to Be Diagnosed with Keratoconus

After my ophthalmologist told me I had Keratoconus, I was shocked that it could ultimately lead to blindness. <u>To not have a known cure acknowledged by the medical field, it was not only hard to imagine, but made me want to look for any alternative</u> treatments that could possibly lessen or eliminate my condition.

The first answer I received from the doctor was that LASIK surgery was <u>not</u> an option because of its dangerous effects on the cornea with Keratoconus. I did some research on the Internet and <u>Dr. Brian was the one doctor that stood out from the rest because</u>

of his accomplishment in finding a solution for Keratoconus and giving people a hope that most people thought impossible.

Before making the trip from New Jersey, I asked Dr. Brian to have a look at my records to see if I was a candidate. Thumbs up! I immediately made reservations and traveled across the country for this amazing breakthrough in modern medicine. It didn't take long for me to finally see again like I had years ago, since the treatment results were immediate.

I would recommend anyone I know who has this disease to Dr. Brian because he is good at what he does and has a great all around staff.

On a final note, **Dr. Brian is not your normal Keratoconus specialist,** however he is someone who keeps you company throughout the whole procedure shaping not only your eyes back to normal but allowing you to stay calm, combining relief with the uneasy tension most patients will expect.

—Giovanni DiMarco, New Jersey
Intacs®, CK and Holcomb C3-R® in 2010

Brian S. Boxer Wachler, MD

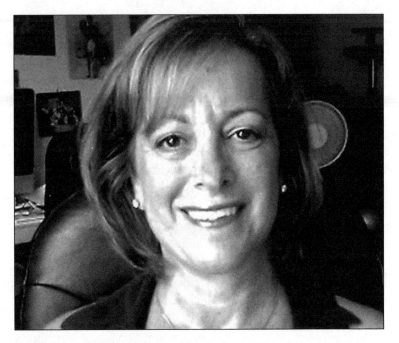

No Cornea Transplant for Me!

I was 26 years old when I was diagnosed with Keratoconus and my ophthalmologist fit me with RGP lenses. As long as I was able to continue wearing RGP lenses, I was not terribly concerned. About ten years later I started having difficulty. My uncorrected eyesight had worsened considerably and <u>I got to the point where corrected I couldn't read street signs until I was very close to them.</u> It was then that MY DOCTOR TOLD ME THAT I WOULD EVENTUALLY NEED A CORNEA TRANSPLANT.

At a family gathering another ten years later a cousin told me about some new research being done to stop the progression of Keratoconus. I mentioned the research to my ophthalmologist.

She had also heard about it and mentioned Dr. Brian. **I went in for a consultation and was blown away by the professionalism of the staff.**

It was determined that I would have Holcomb C3-R® as well as Intacs®. *Both procedures and their recovery were painless and easy.* About a year or so after the procedure, my doctor saw that there had been some progress in the Keratoconus in one of my eyes. I quickly contacted the Boxer Wachler Vision Institute. They brought me back in at no charge and did the Holcomb C3-R® procedure a second time.

Since then, there has been no further progress. I continue to be so grateful that I am able to see (almost) perfectly. I no longer have to dread the eventual necessity of a corneal transplant.

—Laura Gallop, Southern California
Intacs®, CK and Holcomb C3-R® in 2008

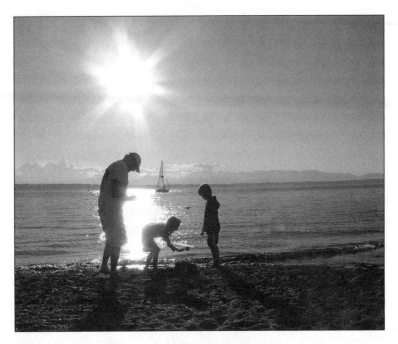

Beating the Hardships of Keratoconus

Every morning the first thing I would barely see was my alarm clock. It was difficult to start every day knowing your vision has changed slightly over night. I visited several specialists and spent lots of time and money on my eyes. I was weary when I was referred to Dr. Brian, thinking he was going to tell me all of the stuff I had tried. I wish I had met him much sooner. I CAN SEE because of him!

—Jeremy Gump, Southern California
Intacs®, CK and Holcomb C3-R® in 2004

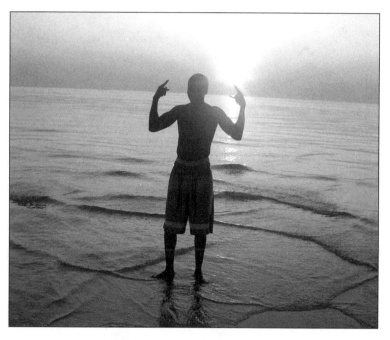

I was Lucky to Find Dr. Brian

When I was diagnosed with Keratoconus **the only solution that I was given was to use hard lenses and wait until I needed a cornea transplant.** I decided to look for my own answers and found Dr. Brian. I got Holcomb C3-R® and Intacs® to improve and stabilize my vision. After three years it's still stable. <u>I have been able to continue with my life without facing the hardships of progressing Keratoconus</u>.

—Fernando Jimeno, Southern California
Intacs® and Holcomb C3-R® in 2009

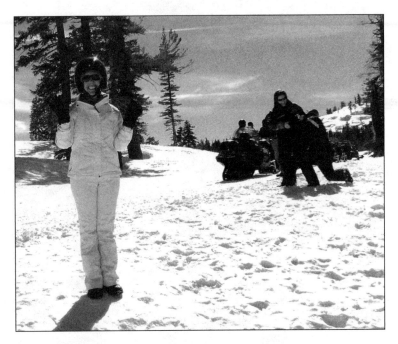

I Followed My Intuition (Gut Feeling), Which Luckily Led Me to Dr. Brian

My journey with Keratoconus began when I was 18 years old. I went to the DMV for a renewal of my driver's license but **I did not pass the vision test.**

I went to my optometrist who saw the beginnings of Keratoconus and referred me to a specialist. The next day I was in with a corneal specialist. I stepped into the world of topographies, bright lights, and various vision tests. <u>Visits to the doctor's office that were at one time yearly, became every 6 months, then every 3 months or so, and then I started becoming a regular, seeing my doctor and contact lens specialist almost weekly</u>.

My doctor talked to me about a corneal transplant. **A cornea transplant just never sat right with me.** I then met an ophthalmologist known to be one of the best in the field, but after my evaluations by him and his team, he strongly recommended a corneal transplant. I called the doctor's office the next morning to sign up on a list to get a corneal transplant, but my intuition was just not calling me to have a transplant.

I **canceled my corneal transplant surgery and started looking into alternate options.** A few days later, I found a doctor who had great success with Keratoconus patients and decided to get his opinion of my eyes and see if he could have some success in fitting me with a comfortable lens that gave me vision. This doctor thought it was time to try some new lenses on my eyes.

We started out with a gas permeable, but as it is inevitable with Keratoconus, it soon was time for a new set of lenses. I did "piggyback" lenses in my eyes for about a year, but then my eyes progressed to the point where I could not wear any lenses whatsoever. At this point more than one doctor was telling me the only option was a cornea transplant and had written me off as a lost cause.

That's when I heard about Steven Holcomb. I SCANNED MY RECORDS AND EMAILED THEM TO DR. BRIAN TO REVIEW. He was willing to take on my case and, after an in-person exam, would decide which procedures would be best for my eyes. I was elated!! I called the next day to book my procedures and trip to LA.

I ended up being eligible for CK, Intacs®, and Holcomb C3-R® and decided to go ahead with all three. During the procedures I was in no pain at all and totally relaxed.

Afterward, the healing and improvements got better month to month. It was awesome! **Halos at night began to decrease dramatically**. A few months post op, I was able to try a soft lenses

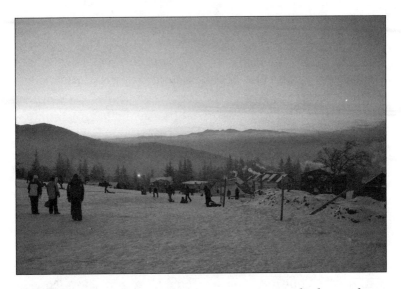

in both eyes that gave me decent vision—<u>my eyes had come leaps and bounds</u>. As my eyes improved more and more, I was able to get even more vision from soft contacts, pretty amazing. Next up is a pair of "more permanent" contact lenses that will give me vision to drive, live, and work fully.

Taking the steps to see Dr. Brian was so worth it. **I am so glad I followed my intuition and took the "out of the box," non-conventional option for my eyes**. <u>It only gets better from here.</u>

—Melissa Spera, Northern California
Intacs®, CK and Holcomb C3-R® in 2010

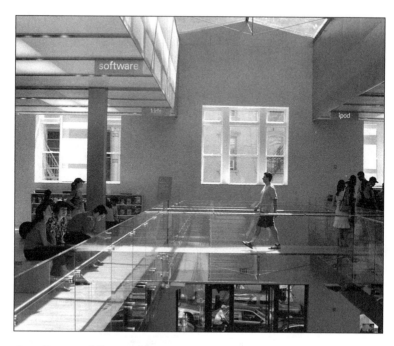

Student Able to Return to School after Keratoconus Treatments

When I was a senior in high school my vision took a turn for the worse. **I was planning on going to college and getting a car, but I couldn't.** Then I got Intacs® and Holcomb C3-R®. <u>My vision has been stable for about 3 years now and I have been able to go back to school and get my driver's license.</u> I know what every patient with Keratoconus goes through, but thanks to Dr. Brian, *Keratoconus doesn't have to control you or your life*.

—Edgar Cabello, Illinois
Intacs®, CK and Holcomb C3-R® in 2009

Brian S. Boxer Wachler, MD

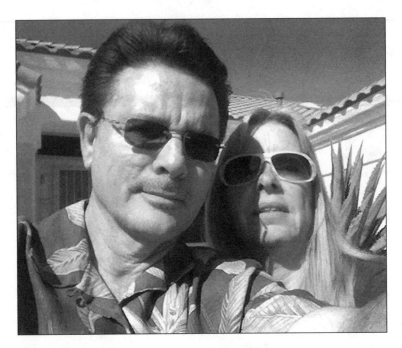

Was Told Intacs® Just a "Gimmick" and Don't Work

I suffered from Keratoconus from the age of 16. I was luckier than most in that I was able to wear RGP lenses for most of my waking day with 20/20 vision. Once the contacts came out I was legally blind. My glasses could not correct my vision with the severe astigmatism.

Unfortunately, right around the age of 46 my eyes started to become drier, they did not produce enough tears and wearing my RGPs for more than just a few hours was intolerable. **My world came crashing down. I am a computer programmer so making a living suddenly became a major concern.**

I visited many cornea specialists across the country and was told almost unanimously I needed transplants. I was aware of Dr. Brian and his ground-breaking work on Intacs®. <u>My very own doctor told me that they were just a gimmick and wouldn't help</u>. <u>With nothing to lose, I visited Dr. Brian anyway</u>. <u>The rest is history</u>.

After Intacs® and later Holcomb C3-R® I now function 100% with just glasses. I NOW SEE 20/20 IN THE RIGHT EYE AND ABOUT 20/40 IN THE LEFT EYE. If there is anyone that has done more to help save vision and make lives easier than Dr. Brian, I would love to meet them.

—Michael White, Texas
Intacs®, CK and Holcomb C3-R® in 2007

Know Your Treatment Options—Have a COMPLIMENTARY Record Review by Dr. Brian

1. Request a copy of your most recent eye exam with color cornea maps from your doctor

2. Describe your situation on a cover sheet with the best phone number and email to contact you

3. Scan and email to: info@boxerwachler.com, or mail to:

Boxer Wachler Vision Institute—KC Records Review
465 N. Roxbury Drive, Suite 902
Beverly Hills, CA 90210

If you have questions, please call us at 310-860-1900. After Dr. Brian's review, we will contact to discuss.

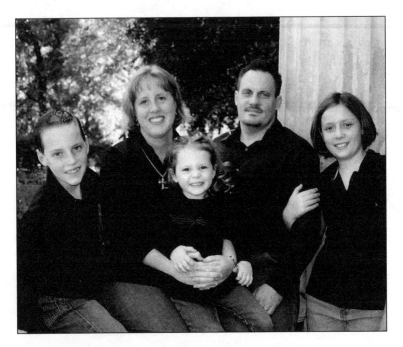

Now I Can Drive My Kids Around and Even Drive at Night!

The first thing I noticed was that I would close one eye every time I tried to read. *I went to several optometrists, but none of them knew what was wrong.* Eventually I was diagnosed with Keratoconus. I tried a series of hard lenses, but I could not tolerate them.

The final reality check for me was when I went to renew my driver's license and FAILED the vision test. I decided to give it one more last ditch effort. I found someone who had developed his own contact lenses specifically for Keratoconus patients. After a lot of pain, I was told that I was headed for a transplant.

It was no longer an option to go uncorrected. I began searching for a better option.

People kept mentioning a doctor in California who was eliminating the need for a transplant. I must have browsed his website four times per week, scrutinizing his research. I decided to call and talk to the doctor to get a feel for why he was doing this. Dr. Brian answered my questions very thoroughly. I sent in my medical records and he said I would likely be a candidate for Intacs®, CK, and Holcomb C3-R®. I scheduled an appointment.

I was in LA for three days and received the Intacs®, Holcomb C3-R®, and CK treatments. I have decided to go without correction because I am tired of messing with contact lenses. I now have 20/30 and 20/40 uncorrected! It's heaven! My life has been completely changed! I am thankful every day that I am able to drive my kids around and can even drive at night!

—Monique Cromis, Texas
Intacs®, CK and Holcomb C3-R® in 2009

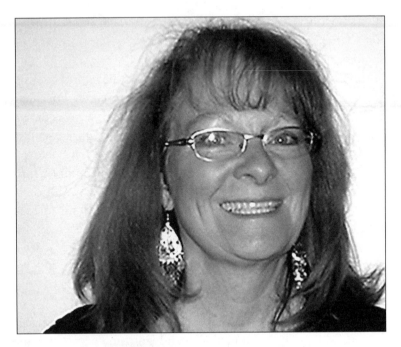

RK Vision Fluctuations Improved— I Have My Life Back!

At the age of 33 years old I went into an eye doctor to determine if I was a candidate for vision correction. Without my contacts I couldn't see where the eye chart was. He did RK (radial keratotomy incision) surgery and my vision was amazingly improved.

By age 43 my vision was fluctuating and I went in to see him again. **He did Lasik on my right eye but the left eye was too unstable.** Glasses and contacts provided limited results.

Now at 54 I learned there were new contact lenses that might help. I called the manufacturer and they referred me to an optometrist. He understood I was having severe vision fluctuations. He saw me Monday morning and had me come back in the afternoon. I explained that tomorrow's fluctuations would not match today's changes. He believed me and had me come in twice a day for a week!

Due to the severe fluctuations my eye doctor didn't believe contacts would work. He asked me to send my records to Dr. Brian to see if Holcomb C3-R® would be an option. Dr. Brian thought Holcomb C3-R® would benefit my vision and slow down the fluctuations. I flew to Beverly Hills, met with Dr. Brian and had Holcomb C3-R®. The procedure was simple to have done! By that evening I noticed my vision was slightly improved. The next day I could read the eye chart better. *Imagine your vision problems going backward,* like unwinding all the years of fluctuations.

NOW YEARS LATER I STILL HAVE JUST ONE PAIR OF GLASSES. I still have some fluctuations but they are very, very minor. *I have my life back.*

—Marcia J., Colorado
Holcomb C3-R® in 2006 (after RK surgery)

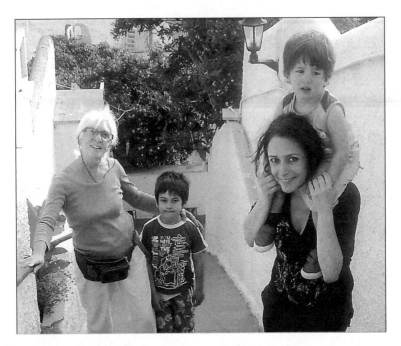

I Am Free of Keratoconus Now and Forever

At age 18 I was diagnosed with Keratoconus. Right away I was given hard contact lenses. Despite them being very painful, I wore them for 15 years. **Then I tried semi-rigid lenses.** They were fantastic. For the first time in 15 years, I could see without pain! But, unknowingly, **I started to develop an allergy to them.**

I had incredible pain, discomfort, and redness all day from the contact lenses and I was forced to stop wearing them. I then heard of a solution called Intacs® that would allow me to wear soft contact lenses. I immediately met with Dr. Brian and set an appointment for the surgery. I didn't have health insurance and had little money at the time, but nothing was going to stop me from doing this.

It all went very well. I was so excited by the genius of Dr. Brian and so trusting in him that I even got Holcomb C3-R®, which was not yet officially FDA approved. **The Intacs® changed my life.** *It went so well, that my eyes were now ready for soft contacts.*

For the first time in more than twenty years I was able to see well without pain in my eyes. My life had been handicapped by Keratoconus, but I AM FREE of it now and forever. **How much better can life get?!!**

—Maude Bonanni, Southern California
Intacs® and Holcomb C3-R® in 2005

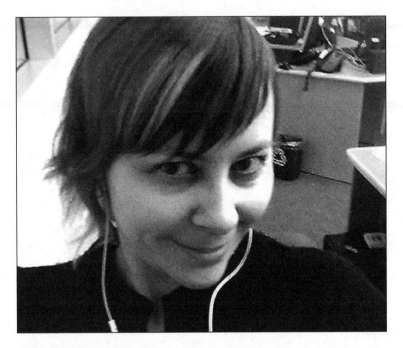

Got My Stubborn Insurance Company to Reimburse Me

I was diagnosed with Keratoconus at age eleven. I wore gas perm contacts through my teen years, but in my 20s I was no longer able to wear gas perm contacts comfortably. **I got by with increasingly stronger glasses and even though I tried lenses**—I'd always end up switching back to wearing my glasses.

Finally, in my early 30s my ophthalmologist told me about Intacs® and Holcomb C3-R® and recommended I see Dr. Brian. It was pretty frustrating knowing that insurance would pay in full for a cornea transplant, but these other treatments that avoid transplant are considered "experimental" by insurance companies.

Dr. Brian advised Intacs® and Holcomb C3-R® as the best means to improve my eyesight (after he reviewed my records).

After the procedures I submitted all paperwork for reimbursement, followed the appeals process and eventually I GOT THE STATE INSURANCE COMMISSIONER TO RULE IN MY FAVOR—I WAS REIMBURSED IN FULL.

It was totally worth it. I am so glad I didn't get a corneal transplant before pursuing all other options.

—Lisa Lindsay, Northern California
Intacs® and Holcomb C3-R® in 2009

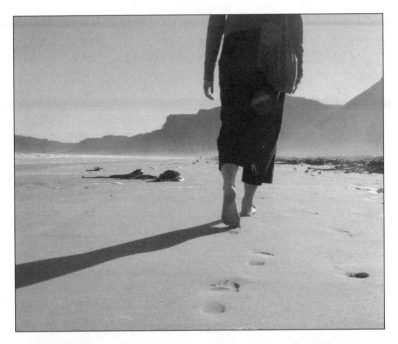

I Had to Find Dr. Brian by Myself—No Glasses Nor Contact Lenses Needed for the Computer

Since being a small child, I can remember that I had to watch TV from a "sideways angle." By the time I was 29 years old, my eyes literally burned every time I sat in front of a computer.

I scheduled a visit to the ophthalmologist who informed me that I had Keratoconus. He then proceeded to refer me to a specialist. The visit was brief and I did not perceive that he had a real interest in my health. I decided **I HAD TO RESEARCH MY OPTIONS BY MYSELF** and educate myself on this condition that was affecting my life and my job.

This is when I found out about Dr. Brian. I read about his practice, I WATCHED THE VERY INFORMATIVE VIDEOS

ON HIS WEBSITE, and found out about the Holcomb C3-R® and Intacs® treatments for Keratoconus. I decided I had found MY own doctor. <u>I could not trust my eyes to anyone but an</u> <u>"EXPERT OF EXPERTS."</u>

I called Dr. Brian's office, forwarded him my records to review, and scheduled an appointment. **Dr. Brian met and exceeded my expectations.** He addressed all my questions, and <u>he did not seem to be in a hurry to leave for his next patient.</u> He informed me in a very detailed manner about every step of the Holcomb C3-R® and Intacs® procedures.

During surgery I felt I was in trusted hands. Needless to say, everything went fine. <u>I was extremely surprised about how</u> <u>immediately I noticed a change in my vision.</u> I can now sit in front of a computer without need for glasses or contacts!

I cannot thank Dr. Brian and his staff enough! I am forever grateful.

—Nallely Cruz, North Carolina
Intacs® and Holcomb C3-R® in 2008

Brian S. Boxer Wachler, MD

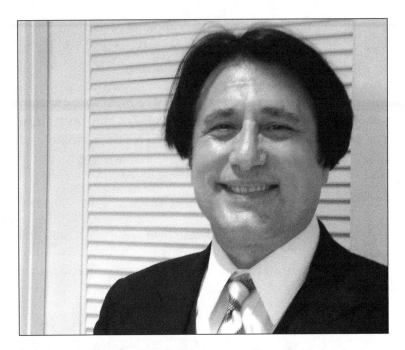

The Procedures Were Simple, Elegant, and Life-Enhancing

During my twenties, I was diagnosed with Keratoconus. For many years, I wore soft toric lenses.

But in the past two years my vision became unstable, making my reading vision less than optimum. Besides the reduced quality of vision, I had become less comfortable in wearing soft lenses.

Subsequently while I was doing online research to find remedies other than the cornea transplant, I came across several articles by and about Dr. Brian.

After an initial inquiry to his Institute and his review of my eye doctor's notes, I made an appointment to visit him. I traveled to Beverly Hills and I received the Holcomb C3-R®, Intacs®, and CK treatments. **The treatments took less than one hour combined.** *Post procedure comfort level was very good.*

It has now been two years since the treatment. I no longer need to wear corrective contact lenses and my reading ability is excellent!

Because of my profession, I deal with a lot of new technologies that come out of laboratories and go through commercialization stage in the healthcare field. <u>The combined procedures I went through, in my view, represent science at its best: simple, elegant, and life-enhancing</u>.

Congratulations to Dr. Brian and his fine staff for operationalizing an array of advanced scientific discoveries. THEIR DAZZLING SCIENCE IS MATCHED WITH EQUALLY IMPRESSIVE PATIENT CARE. The staff at the Boxer Wachler Vision Institute are indeed excellent and their professionalism and friendliness are truly exemplary.

—Nasser Arshadi, Missouri
Intacs®, CK and Holcomb C3-R® in 2010

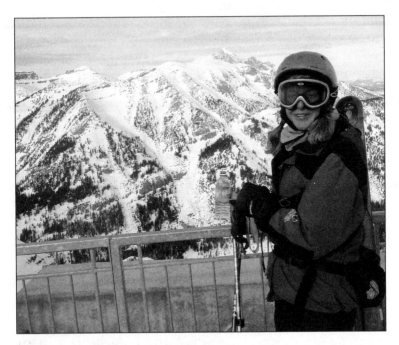

Myth Busted: Hard Contact Lenses DON'T Slow Down Keratoconus

I was diagnosed with Keratoconus in 1981. I was pregnant with my first child and was very frustrated because it took many months to get fitted for contact lenses. *I remember that when my son was born, I couldn't see whether he was a boy or a girl.*

I finally got fitted and was told that in 40 years I would have to have a cornea transplant. Forty years seemed like an eternity so I went on with my life and was very blessed to have comfortable hard contacts.

Twenty nine years later when I had my annual visit with my eye doctor, I was reminded how serious my disease was. That 29 years went by fast! **My eye doctor in New Mexico referred me to Dr. Brian's website for Holcomb C3-R®.**

I became VERY FRIGHTENED when I learned the truth about hard contact lenses: **hard contacts do NOT slow the Keratoconus progression** and that <u>I could go blind without treatment</u>.

I immediately researched my options and arranged treatment. After Dr. Brian's analysis of my medical records, he advised CK and Holcomb C3-R® with the goal of better vision with the RGP contacts.

My optometrist is very impressed! I had CK done along with Holcomb C3-R®, and she can see the positive changes in my cornea.

I am so thankful!

—Diane Smith, New Mexico
CK and Holcomb C3-R® in 2010

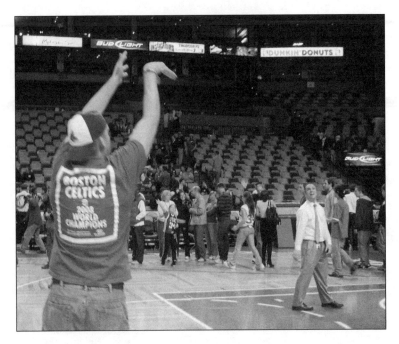

Found Out About Dr. Brian During Olympic Coverage of Steven Holcomb

When I was 21 years old I went to the DMV to get my license renewed and was SHOCKED when I couldn't see anything. I'd had no idea it was that bad.

The next day <u>I was diagnosed with Keratoconus and told that a cornea transplant would be the only way to cure this</u>. So about a month passed and I was still mulling over all the decisions and I ended up watching the Olympics. **At one point they were interviewing Steven Holcomb of the U.S. Bobsled team. He was talking about how he used to have Keratoconus and his career was basically over until he went to Dr. Brian who fixed it.**

I immediately went to the computer, looked at Dr. Brian's website, and sent in my eye exam information for him to evaluate. About 3 months later I flew to California and ended up getting the Holcomb C3-R®, Intacs®, and CK treatments. My vision remained blurry for about 2 days, but once it wore off <u>I couldn't believe I had been living my life through the eyes I used to have. The difference was astounding</u>!

So about a month and a half after we got back I went to see my regular doctor. He was so shocked. After we all sat down I read the eye chart. I could see the 6th row down, where before I couldn't even see the Big E! I'D GONE FROM 20/500 VISION TO 20/50 VISION UNCORRECTED!

I will never forget what Dr. Brian and his staff did for me and how happy and blessed I truly am.

—Steve Mavilia, Massachusetts
Intacs®, CK and Holcomb C3-R® in 2010

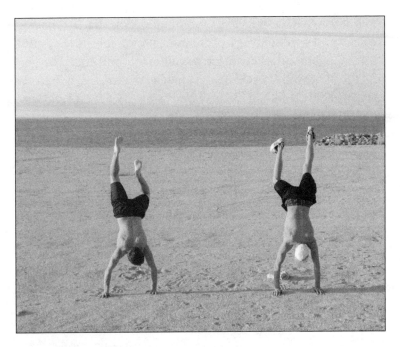

My Child Can Now Live Life as a Normal Teenager

My son, Chad, had always enjoyed playing sports and video games, like most young boys his age. But when he was about 12 years old, he began having trouble. Thinking he might need glasses, I set up an eye exam.

His doctor diagnosed Chad with Keratoconus. **The only option I had was to fit Chad with special contacts**, but I felt we needed to wait a year because he needed to have a better sense of responsibility first. At this time I really did not know much about the disease. NO ONE TOLD ME HIS EYES COULD DETERIORATE AS FAST AS THEY DID.

Later he was unable to wear the lenses and was told his vision loss had progressed. *Our doctor said we needed to start thinking about corneal transplants.* Suddenly I realized the decisions that would affect him the rest of his life were suddenly thrust upon us.

I did not want to think about having to do corneal transplants on my 16 year old. Then the doctor here in Ohio mentioned Dr. Brian. I had never heard of Holcomb C3-R®, but after reading about what Dr. Brian had done, I decided Chad needed to see him and I sent his records in for a review.

The Intacs®, CK, and C3-R® treatments that Dr. Brian did changed my son's life. With everything that was done Chad can finally reach for his dreams and live a life as a normal teenager. The decision we made was hard, but I feel we could not have made a better choice with the help of Dr. Brian.

—Teresa Gravesmill, Chad's Mother, Ohio
Intacs®, CK and Holcomb C3-R® in 2010

Know Your Treatment Options—Have a COMPLIMENTARY Record Review by Dr. Brian

1. Request a copy of your most recent eye exam with color cornea maps from your doctor

2. Describe your situation on a cover sheet with the best phone number and email to contact you

3. Scan and email to: info@boxerwachler.com, or mail to:

Boxer Wachler Vision Institute—KC Records Review
465 N. Roxbury Drive, Suite 902
Beverly Hills, CA 90210

If you have questions, please call us at 310-860-1900.
After Dr. Brian's review, we will contact to discuss.

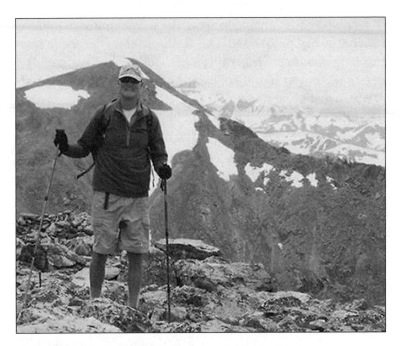

Became Intolerant to Contact Lenses and Needed a Solution

Prior to Dr. Brian treating my Keratoconus, my vision was at best 20/25 in the left eye and 20/40 in the right eye. My local ophthalmologist had me wear "Saturn" soft contacts with a gas permeable lens in the center. This solution worked for a few years, but eventually I developed conjunctivitis in my eyes.

After that, I tried the gas permeable contacts, but found them uncomfortable. *I like to ski, ride my mountain bike, hike and play golf.* Glasses worked for me most of the time at home and at work, but <u>nothing is worse than to be skiing and have the glasses fog up or be out on my bike and have it start raining</u>. Not much fun.

I took the next step and forwarded my local eye doctor's records in to Dr. Brian to review.

I had the Holcomb C3-R®, CK, and Intacs® treatments with Dr. Brian and a few months later I went back for the Visian ICL™ procedure. Now **I see 20/20 uncorrected with both eyes.** My close vision is pretty good; I can see my computer monitor and dashboard in my car and generally can read in good lighting conditions (unless the print is really small) without reading glasses.

The first time I went skiing after the Visian ICL™—IT WAS INCREDIBLE. <u>I could actually see where I was going and not do it by feel alone.</u> <u>No more foggy glasses on the slopes!</u>

—Scott Macdonald, Colorado
Intacs®, CK, Holcomb C3-R® and Visian ICL in 2010

Brian S. Boxer Wachler, MD

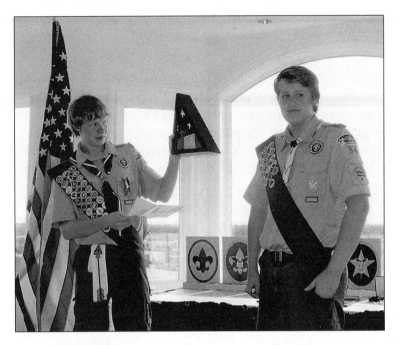

For the First Time, I Now Can See in 3-D

When I was 12 years old, my vision got blurry. My mom tried getting me glasses, but that didn't really help my vision so I didn't wear them.

A year later, the eye doctor diagnosed me with Keratoconus. He said I would need to wear contacts to correct my vision and I was fitted for lenses that day. *A month later, after a lot of research, my mom explained to me what Keratoconus really was and that there were some treatments available that could save my eyesight from getting worse.*

Neither one of us was even told that I could someday lose my vision or need a corneal transplant. IT WAS A GOOD

78

THING WE HAD THE INTERNET. **We learned about Dr. Brian.** Through the Internet she found out about the Boxer Wachler Vision Institute and contacted them about the possibility of getting the Holcomb C3-R® treatment for me.

After getting a second opinion from a corneal specialist, my parents decided that getting the treatment right away by Dr. Brian was best. He reviewed my medical records and recommended Intacs®, CK and Holcomb C3-R®. We made the trip out to California to get the treatment.

I had the Holcomb C3-R®, CK, and Intacs® procedures. I was scared about the treatment and what to expect, but everyone was so nice and explained everything very well.

Now it's two years later and my vision is totally stable, so the Holcomb C3-R® is doing its job. I have a good chance of keeping the vision I now have. I have new contacts now, and, *for the first time, I have been able to watch a 3-D movie at the IMAX theatre and ACTUALLY see it in 3-D!*

—Robert Goes, Idaho
Intacs®, CK and Holcomb C3-R® in 2010

Brian S. Boxer Wachler, MD

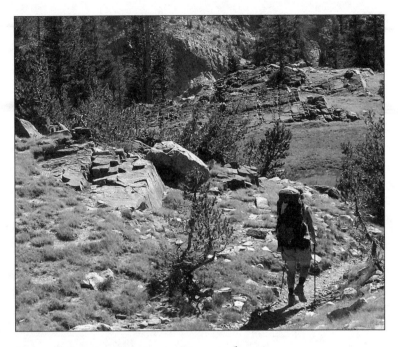

Saved from a Cornea Transplant

About 20 years ago, when I was diagnosed with Keratoconus, the only option was a cornea transplant. **Eventually, I was considered nearly blind and "needed" a transplant.** Research revealed an alternative: Intacs®. After careful consideration, I underwent the procedure. Intacs® WAS PAINLESS and successful, and <u>the skillful hands of Dr. Brian improved my vision and saved me from a cornea transplant.</u>

—David Mathies, Southern California
Intacs® in 2004

ABOUT Brian S. Boxer Wachler, MD—
"the KERATOCONUS GURU"

Dr. Brian is regarded as one of the top leaders in the sub-specialty of Keratoconus. His role as the "doctor's doctor" has been earned through his unwavering integrity and broad expertise. He is often consulted by other eye surgeons who need assistance with challenging patients or by patients who need repairs for previous Keratoconus surgery. His peers come to him when they need eye surgery.

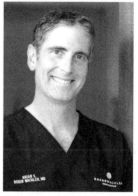

"Dr. Brian" S. Boxer Wachler

As well as being Board Certified by the <u>American Board of Ophthalmology,</u> he was elected to the <u>International Refractive Surgery Club</u> (IRSC), a leadership society of the world's best refractive surgeons. Prior to founding the Boxer Wachler Vision Institute in Beverly Hills, California, he was director of the UCLA Laser Refractive Center at the Jules Stein Eye Institute.

Dr. Brian pioneered the use of Intacs® for Keratoconus in the United States in 1999 and since then has performed several thousand Keratoconus procedures on patients from all over the world. He published the largest study on Intacs® treatment for Keratoconus, which the FDA used for their approval of Intacs® for Keratoconus. Due to his pioneering work, Intacs® is now officially recognized as a treatment for Keratoconus.

Dr. Brian was the first doctor in the U.S., Canada, South America, Asia, Latin America, and Europe (except Germany) to perform corneal collagen crosslinking. *After using corneal collagen crosslinking since 2003,* **he has the LONGEST EXPERIENCE with it than any other doctor in the world (except Germany).** He invented the non-invasive, 1 day recovery C3-R® Crosslinking System in 2003.

He is the Chief Editor of the landmark book *Modern Management of Keratoconus,* which was first published in 2008. This is one of the most detailed and widely used books in the training of doctors around the world. This is the **"FIRST"** book to address alternatives to cornea transplant.

He customizes Keratoconus procedures for each patient to stop the devastating loss of vision, while actually improving vision and quality of life.

Dr. Brian received the 2010 Jules Stein Living Tribute Award for **performing the vision saving C3-R® crosslinking treatment on U.S. Olympic bobsled driver Steve Holcomb.** This restored his vision, enabling him to win the gold metal at the 2010 Winter Olympics in Vancouver—the first for the United States bobsled team in 62 years. Subsequently Dr. Brian renamed the procedure Holcomb C3-R® Crosslinking System in honor of Steven Holcomb who brought worldwide attention to this vision preserving treatment.

Many of Dr. Brian's accomplishments, publications and commendations can be found on the Internet. Try entering "brian boxer wachler" into your favorite search engine.

Professional Experience

- Boxer Wachler Vision Institute, *Director (present position)*
- Complications Repair Clinic for referred patients, *Director (present position)*
- UCLA Laser Refractive Center, *Director*

- Refractive Surgery Resident and Fellowship Training, Jules Stein Eye Institute
- Refractive Surgery Clinic, University of Kansas Medical Center, *Director*

Education and Training

- University of Kansas Medical Center, *Fellowship in Refractive and Corneal Surgery*
- Saint Louis University Eye Institute, *Residency in Ophthalmology*
- Dartmouth Medical School, New Hampshire, *Doctor of Medicine*
- Edinburgh University, Scotland, *Rotary International Scholar*
- University of California, Los Angeles, *Bachelor of Science in Psychobiology*

Honors and Awards

- Jules Stein Living Tribute Award for inventing Holcomb C3-R® Crosslinking System
- Secretariat Award, American Academy of Ophthalmology
- Top Fifty Opinion Leaders in Cataract and Refractive Surgery
- Voted one of the Best Doctors in America
- Voted one of America's Top Ophthalmologists, Consumer Research Council of America
- Career Senior Achievement Award, American Academy of Ophthalmology
- International Society of Refractive Surgery (ISRS) Annual Symposia, *Vice-Chair*
- Indian Intraocular Implant and Refractive Surgery Society, *Gold Medal Award for Career Scientific Contributions*

- Distinguished National Ophthalmologist Award
- Elected to the <u>International Refractive Surgery Club</u> (IRSC),
- Bausch & Lomb Pharmaceuticals, *Travel Grant for Young Investigators Award*
- Saint Louis University Eye Institute, *Research Award*
- ISRS, Resident Travel Scholarship

Thought Leadership

Dr. Brian is a thought leader at the forefront of Keratoconus treatments. He is trusted by patients, colleagues and by the state and federal government. The Department of Defense and United States Army recently honored Dr. Brian for his scientific contributions.

- Intacs® clinical trials, *FDA investigator*
- Phakic intraocular lenses (implantable contact lenses) clinical trials, *FDA investigator*

Dr. Brian plays a key role in the global field of vision correction. His work has changed the way surgeons perform vision correction procedures.

- Established industry LASIK guidelines to prevent halos and glare and decrease Keratoconus risk
- Widely published in the scientific literature for innovations in the field
- Pioneer of Intacs® for Keratoconus
- <u>Center for Keratoconus</u>, *Board of Directors*
- Communications Committee for the <u>International Society of Refractive Surgery</u>, the global organization of more than 2,500 cornea/refractive surgeons, *Chairman*

Media Appearances

Dr. Brian has had a considerable number of media appearances as the featured expert in local and national media. Here's a few of them:

Television:

The Today Show, The Doctors—Dr. Phil Production, *EXTRA, Good Day LA,* and *Dr. Drew's LifeChangers, NBC Nightly News, NBC News, ABC News, CBS News, FOX News, CNN News,* and PBS' *American Health Journal.*

Radio:

National Public Radio (NPR), KNX News, KFWB News

Press:

Los Angeles Times, New York Times, Wall Street Journal, Time Magazine, Newsweek, US News and World Report, USA Today, AOL Health, Shape Magazine, and *Forbes.*

Dr. Brian performed LIVE eye surgery on NBC'S Today Show in front of millions of viewers. After that "heart-pounding" experience, he made a documentary film because of the unbelievable events that occurred BEHIND THE SCENES. **To watch this very entertaining movie that was even shown in a film festival, please go to www.boxerwachler.com/movie.**

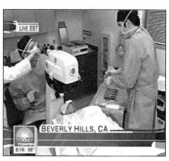

You won't believe what happened behind the scenes on the Today Show.

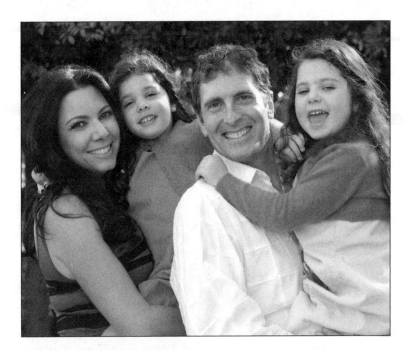

More about Dr. Brian

Dr. Brian has been married for 19 years to Selina, whom he met in college at summer camp where they were counselors. He refers to her as his "summer camp sweetheart."

They have two fraternal twin daughters, born in 2006. Dr. Brian is a "family man" and takes every Monday afternoon off from the office to pick up his girls from school.

Dr. Brian gives back to the community and supports a number of non-profit organizations, including Boys and Girls Clubs of America, Make-a-Wish Foundation, Wounded Warrior Project, among others. He founded the Giving Vision charity and Homeless Not Sockless program which donates fresh, new socks to the homeless.

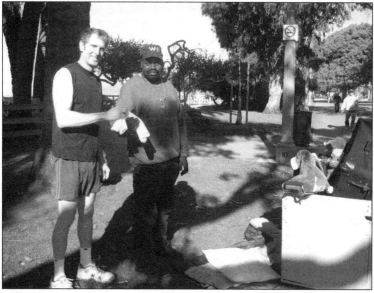

Dr. Brian giving new socks to the homeless in Los Angeles as part of his "Homeless Not Sockless" program.

As a former college athlete on the crew (rowing) teams at UCLA and Edinburgh University, Dr. Brian still enjoys rowing and competing in local and national rowing competitions. He recently won the Bronze medal at the United States Masters National Rowing Championships.

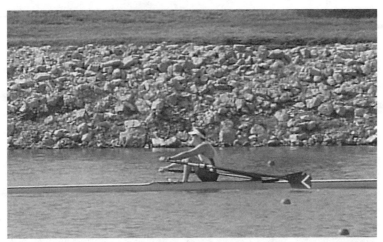

Dr. Brian racing in the finals at the U.S. Masters National Rowing Championships.

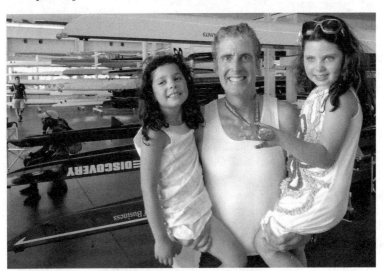

With the bronze medal and two "gold medals" in each arm!

THE RACE

by Beth Barnes, mother of Ian Barnes, Ohio, Holcomb C3-R® and Intacs® in 2012

BEFORE THE SUN AWAKENS
AND EAGLES TAKE THEIR FLIGHT
YOU WILL FIND HIM IN HIS SCULLY
THE MAN WHO GIVES BACK SIGHT

THE DARKNESS STARTS TO FADE TO LIGHT
THE MIST BEGINS TO LIFT
THE BEGINNING OF ANOTHER DAY
TO USE HIS SPECIAL GIFT

HE WORKS WITH SUCH PRECISION
SIDE BY SIDE WITH HIS TALENTED CREW
TO WIN THIS PRECIOUS RACE OF SIGHT
TO SEE THE WORLD BRAND NEW

AND WHEN AT DUSK
THE SUN DOES SET
ANOTHER RACE IS WON
TOMORROW IS ANOTHER DAY
HIS WORK IS NOT YET DONE . . .

COMPLIMENTARY KERATOCONUS DVD OR BOOK!

There are three ways to claim your complimentary Keratoconus DVD or book.

To receive your complimentary DVD of *MODERN MANAGEMENT OF KERATOCONUS* or Dr. Brian's latest book *MASTERY OF COLLAGEN CROSSLINKING FOR KERATOCONUS*, please either:

Please fax this form to: 310-860-1902, or

Mail this form to: 465 N. Roxbury Drive, Suite 902, Beverly Hills, CA 90210, or

Call 310-860-1900

YES! I would like to receive my complimentary copy of

(PLEASE CHECK ONLY ONE)

❏ DVD *MODERN MANAGEMENT OF KERATOCONUS*

❏ Dr. Brian's latest book *MASTERY OF COLLAGEN CROSSLINKING FOR KERATOCONUS*

_____

First name   Last Name

_____

Address

_____

City/State/Zip Code

_____

Primary e-mail